ABOUT THIS BOOK

It is safe to say that the majority of people around the world cannot afford good psychotherapy. At $80 to $185 per hour, many are not getting the help they need to live the life they imagined. That's why I have written DIY Therapies: Affordable and Effective. I'm a published therapeutic innovator with a desire to see that no one is left without the psychological help they need simply because they can't afford it. DIY Therapies: Affordable and Effective includes three, easy to follow, problem-solving techniques for relief from chronic pain, depression and obsessive thinking. DIY Therapies: Affordable and Effective is about taking control of your health and your future: about living the life you imagine.

CONTENTS

FORWARD

Don't let the simplicity of these therapies cause you to think they are not effective. Simplicity is one of the keys to effective, life-altering therapy. As an innovator of therapeutic approaches, I endeavour to hone down each therapy to its essential components. I don't like to waste anyone's time. There is really no need for week after week visits to an expensive psychologist, therapist or counsellor. If a therapist's technique and ability are good, a client should gain insight and relief after the first visit.

Ninety per cent of psychotherapeutic healing comes from within the client, not from the downloading efforts of a therapist. This set of three innovations has been created to help not only produce relief from psychological or physiological problems, but help move people in the direction of authenticity. In other words, you will find relief from depression, chronic pain and obsessive thinking and, in the process, you will move closer to the knowledge of who you are – closer to your identity.

Most psychological problems are created as a result of a movement away from the knowledge of Self. This movement is often toward an erroneous understanding of identity. These unhelpful ideas about whom one is are most often heaped upon an individual as a result of cultural ideas, social norms, systems of thought, media, well-meaning family and significant others. Physical pain is not much different than psychological pain in that it moves people away from authenticity via cultural conscripts and social ideas of strong and weak. The loss of an ability to remain congruent with these ideas (however biased or patriarchal they are) is the ground of more physiological pain and, on top of this, the creation of psychological pain. These therapies are intended to bring you into greater contact with your authentic self. All therapy should have this goal. This movement toward authenticity is an essential component of healing.

I hope you ready yourself for what is written herein. Before you begin to read this book, invite hope and possibility in. Most of all, don't race through it. Each part will require your deep thinking about what is really happening in your life and mind and what you really want. You will also need rest. I suggest you rest between each part of each individual therapy. You'll not gain much by reading this book cover to cover like a novel. It is a therapeutic book and ninety percent of the problem solving is going to come from within you. So slow down, trust your inner wisdom, your ability to heal and change, and welcome what comes from your subconscious.

"When one door closes another door opens, but we so often look so long and so regretfully upon the closed door, that we do not see the ones which open for us."
Alexander Graham Bell

To the above quote, my mother often added, "Yes, but it can be hell in the hallway!" Through this book, you are soon to be on your way into and back out of the hallway.

Laurel Phillips MSW RSW
Narrative Therapist and Community Worker

DIY RELIEF FROM DEPRESSION

Many people spend weeks or months in therapy trying to figure out what the problem is. Once this discovery has been made, people spend the majority of their time and money trying to get rid of it. Most have no idea why they are depressed, and they very much dislike having to take medication daily to keep from coming apart at the seams. The problem you have right now is about to become a door to the solution. Once you have a good understanding of the purposes of the problem, no other problem will EVER seem the same to you.

The purposes of any problem are:
1. To act as a signpost, pointing the way to a solution and helping you find your way to wholeness.
2. To help you better know yourself.

A problem's only reason for living is to help you live the life you want. This is important to understand. The problem is in your life to help you live the life you imagine. It is present to show you that something is wrong in your life. It would never be present if there weren't some part of life that was not working well for you.

When we experience a psychological change, such as the onset of depression, we automatically assign this occurrence with a quality of either good or bad. It is just part of the human experience to perceive something and then make a snap judgment on it, but that quality assignation is not necessarily correct. The quality of either good or bad that we assign to experiences emerges from what we have been taught. These teachings come via culture, family, social systems of thought, and through all sorts of avenues. The quality we assign our experience is often part of group thinking.

For example, if women in your culture believe that being fat is bad then overweight women might be thought of as being lazy or ugly or deficient in will. And you, by cultural default, are likely to carry this thought pattern as well, assigning these attributes to all overweight women. However, if you are African and live somewhere on the African subcontinent, where food is scarce, and a heavy set woman appears in your village, you are likely to think that she is wealthy and intelligent. Likewise, if you're a North American and a new neighbour moves in next to you with three young wives, you will probably always look sideways at him, wondering how he became such a low-life who takes advantage of women and judging his young wives as stupid or naive. However, if you were Tibetan woman and lived on the Tibetan Plateau and your closest neighbour was a woman who married three brothers, you'd feel a sense of happiness for her, perhaps even pride if you also have three brothers in your home that are your husbands.

I hope you are you beginning to see that the quality we assign any experience is something given to us by those in our culture who previously assigned quality. I am not suggesting that depression is good or bad. I am only opening up a small window to the possibility that this event, this experience of depression, can be used as a catalyst for healing. Depression does not need to take you out if you let it take you to higher ground.

Years ago, when my son was ten and I was a single parent raising him alone, we had a visit from a couple of Jehovah's Witnesses. A conversation ensued in which we debated Satan's purpose. I was not sure what I felt Satan's purpose was. The JW women felt Satan's purpose was to punish bad humans. At that moment, my ten-year-old son came whizzing down the hallway from his bedroom, coming to a sliding stop in his socked feet and said, "Satan's purpose is to turn your face toward God." All three of us were gobsmacked and silent for a good thirty seconds. Then I broke our silence and said, "Out of the mouth of babes".

By following this DIY guide, you're going to use the problem to discover what's wrong. The problem of depression is here to help you find out what important and cherished ways of living are not able to have full expression in your life.

A breakdown of this therapeutic process:
1. Naming the problem.
2. Determining the influence of the problem.
3. Justifying its influence.
    Rest
4. Stepping toward the solution.
    Rest
5. Identity markers: Clues to who you really are.
    Belief statements and values
6. Who are You?
    How Did You Come to Live With depression?
    Side Note: A Few Words About Medication
7. Bringing it all together.

Get a pen and some paper, or better yet, a journal. To achieve success, you're going to need to answer a few questions. Be honest and fearless about your answers.

Naming the problem

Take a few minutes to find a name for the problem. You might be happy with the name, "depression". Or you might want to use some other descriptor such as "The Black Cloud" or "Misery".

Find a name you are comfortable with.

Write that name in your journal by completing this statement: The name of the problem is _____.

Whatever you do, DON'T STOP, even if the going gets tough. Difficult goals are always worth a little struggle. Winston Churchill once said, "If you're going through hell, keep going." And, "Never, never, never give up." Churchill also suffered the influence of a depression he called the "Black Dog".

Use your imagination to visualise the problem. Close your eyes and imagine what this depression (or whatever you named the problem) looks like? Is it big or little? What colour is it? Does it have a distinct shape, like an animal or human, or is it more amorphous or shapeless? I want you to make the problem small enough to fit it into the palm of your hand. Next, use your imagination to put the problem into a glass jar and seal it with a tight-fitting lid. Using your imagination to change the size of the problem will not necessarily change its effect on life. For some, however, this does alter the problem.

Take some time to think about what life is like when you hold the problem in a jar. Does using your imagination this way feel like you have a bit more control over the problem? For most people, using their imagination to create a different perspective of the problem allows them to feel some immediate relief.

Determining the influence of the problem

It is now time to write about the influence this problem has had in your life. How has this problem influenced your relationships with others? How has it influenced your life or the life you want to live? How has the problem influenced your relationship with yourself, you're children, spouse, partner. . ? Are you more or less confident around the problem? Has the problem affected your job career? Is the problem threatening your goals and dreams? In your journal, write down at least five ways that the problem has or is influencing life. If you want, use the following statement:

The problem of _____ has affected my _____ in the following ways _____.

Justifying the influence of the problem

Justify your evaluation of the influence that this problem is having on your life by answering the following question:

Are you OK with the influence this problem is having on life? Yes or No?

Keep in mind that the influence might not be negative all the time. It might be that the depression allows you to spend time alone and you like to be alone or, it might be that the depression causes you to turn off your phone, but you never really liked talking on the phone. Sometimes, the problem has a combination of both good and bad influences.

Write your justification answer(s) in your journal using the following statement:

I am not ok with the influence the problem has on my life because it causes me to _____.

If the problem has had some positive influence on life, complete the next statement as well.

I am OK with the influence the problem has on my life because it allows me to _____.

Write down at least five statements about the problem's influence on life.

Rest

I realize that you may be tired with the negative influence this problem has had on your life and that you might be anxious to get rid of it so you can enjoy living your life without its influence. I don't blame you for wanting to get this over and done with, but rushing through this DIY is not going to give you the kind of results that taking your time will. Taking your time with this DIY is going to help you ingest the material, allowing it to settle in and create new ways of thinking. Going at a slower pace is a kinder approach to change and it allows for insight to emerge.

Some change that results from therapy is instantaneous. This kind of change is the result of insight. Insight comes from a universal source and, when you receive an insight, life is altered instantly. Insight produces the 'AHA' effect and it marks epiphany moments. There is no need to cogitate information in an attempt to produce change when insight is present.

Taking your time with this DIY and meditating on the ideas that are surfacing through answering the questions can produce insight. Insight is another reason for you to rest and take this slowly.

Stepping toward the solution

Whatever you wrote after the word 'because' holds a key to solving this problem. You are now going to mine those five statements for solutions. Those solutions are going to be found in the values, beliefs, commitments for living, goals and dreams that those five statements express.

A value is a word that describes what is important to you.

A belief is a statement or idea built around a value.

A commitment for living is a way of life that you believe is important.

A goal is an achievement on the horizon that you are working toward.

A dream is the big picture of life - what you hope to accomplish. It envelops and reflects many important ways of life.

Write those five (or more) statements out again. This time begin just after the word 'because'.

Example #1: "I am not OK with the influence of depression because it keeps me from going out with my family." You only need this part of the above statement that comes after the word because. "It keeps me from going out with my family."

Example #2: "I'm not OK with depression (or whatever you named the problem) because I have to take medication and it makes me too tired to complete goals." You could mine this statement for two values or beliefs. They are: "I have to take medication and it makes me too tired to complete goals."

Example #3: I'm OK with depression because it gives me a reason to not go out and hang with people." "It gives me a reason to not go out and hang with people."

You're not quite at a succinct list of values and beliefs, but rather, you have statements that require further mining. Once you have the above statements, however, you have only a short distance to go to identify the values and beliefs that constitute who you are. These values and beliefs will be used to undermine depression and increase authenticity.

Rest

Are you remembering to take breaks? Try to see times of rest as an important part of the healing and growth process. You wouldn't have surgery on your knee and not rest it up for several weeks. Likewise, changing the way you think needs time to settle in and become not just new thoughts, but new ways of life.

Identity markers: Clues to who you really are

Couched within the statements above are identity markers. These markers tell everyone you meet who you are and what you stand for; what's important to you. These markers are your values, beliefs, commitments for living, goals and dreams.

Using example #1 (I'm making this up as I go)follow the steps below to help you define important identity markers:

Step 1: Write out the statement in full. "I am not OK with the influence of depression because it keeps me from going out with my family."

Step 2: Write out the part that comes after the word 'because'. "it keeps me from going out with my family."

The problem points to something that is important to you, but that is not able to have expression in life at this time. It speaks of the important belief, value or commitment that you hold precious and that needs expression. The statement above, "It keeps me from going out with my family", could be about the importance of family, time, freedom or life. Only you know the value or belief that is couched in the statement. To retrieve it, you'll need to trust yourself and listen for what comes from deep inside. Investigate each statement you wrote for the important beliefs you hold about life.

A belief that might be couched in the statement, "It keeps me from going out with my family", might be, I should be able to go where I want when I want.
The value that is producing this belief might be 'freedom' or 'freedom to choose'.

You'll find a very extensive list of values to help you locate what is important to you in the appendix at the end of this book.

Don't get hung up on finding the precise value that emerges from your belief statements. That is not the most important part of this exercise. Simply take what emerges for you and write it down. You'll find out soon whether it belongs or not when we look for common threads in your discoveries.

Belief statements and values

You are going to collect five belief statements and five values that are reflected in your 'because' statements. This can be challenging. Countless people struggle to describe their values and beliefs. Some people didn't know they had values and beliefs until I helped them uncover these in therapy sessions. Through these investigations, we are digging deeper into what makes YOU, YOU. This work is akin to an archaeological dig into your life. All you need to do is take your 'because' statements and translate them into belief statements. It might sound difficult, but it's not, especially if you can trust what comes up while you think about these statements.

Time and time again, when I investigate these statements with clients, I know when we have found accurate values and beliefs when I hear them say something similar to this, "Well, this might seem odd but ... " Often, when a person is suffering from depression they have limited insight into what's important to them. This is a strong reason for depression's presence. People are moved away from values, beliefs and important ways of living slowly, over a lifetime, through adherence to cultural demands or through tragic or traumatic experiences. The discovery of important ways of living brings insight moments that often contribute to knowledge about authenticity. In other words, clients are tickled to find out that they hold certain values that they were never able to define or articulate in the past.

These values and beliefs were always present and the problem was always pointing in their direction. The degree of the problem, the depth of it or the badness of it is an indication that a person is tightly holding onto their values and beliefs. The more troubling the problem is for a client, the more resistance or tight-holding is being demonstrated.

Here are a few more examples:

#1. "I'm not OK with depression (or whatever you called it) because I feel ugly when it is here."
I feel ugly when it is here."
Feeling ugly is the problem that depression is pointing to.
This is a problem because of a value, belief or commitment to liv-

ing that needs expression.
Belief = I am not ugly. I am beautiful.
Value = Beauty (or self-esteem, or self-love).

#2.
"I'm not OK with depression (or whatever you called it) because it keeps me from playing with my kids."
"It keeps me from playing with my kids."
Belief = my kids are important
Value = family (or children, or . . .)

Collect five belief statements (ex. "My kids are important") and five single-word values (ex. Children) and write them in your journal.

When I say that we hold a value, what I mean is that we place high regard on that value. If you value beauty then beauty is valuable to you. It is important. Your values and beliefs describe WHO YOU ARE. As you might be noticing, these investigations are quickly becoming about identity. Knowing who you are, your identity, leads to authentic living. Furthermore, living an authentic life is an important part of knowing what you should do with your life. Authenticity, therefore, leads to purpose.

The beliefs and values that you uncovered through this exercise describe who you are. They are a small collection of indicators that tell the world what makes life important to you or what makes life worth living. They speak about what you stand for and what you are not willing to accept. I can assure you that there is nothing more powerful, that is an important contributor to an excellent life than knowing who we are. Identity is everything.

By now, through this DIY therapy, you have come to know about important values and beliefs you hold by investigating what depression was pointing to in terms of important ways of living that were being suppressed and that desperately needed expression. Lack of expression was causing depression. You were holding these important ways back, but you were also fiercely protecting them because of the degree of importance they held for you. Many people hold back or suppress important ways of being in service to conformity. They have been convinced that it is more important to conform to social or cultural ideas about good and bad, right and wrong, strong and weak and so on because they have made the assumption that to be authentic would mean they would be rejected or unwanted; left alone and abandoned. These made up cultural/social ideas contradicted what you valued so, to avoid the threat of abandonment, you opted to hide important aspects of yourself in favour of being someone else; some created person. Depression has come on the scene of life to help you understand that you MUST live life according to who you are, despite the fear and threats that your thinking might present. Try to think of the fear and threats as only being generated from cultural ideas. Honestly, that's really all it is.

Who are you?

How did these values come to be important to you? How did these beliefs and values come to be such an important part of your identity? Sit back and take a few minutes to let the values and belief that you have discovered sink in. Re-read your list and look for values that are similar. Group these similar values together. Next, we'll search your personal archives for reasons why these are important. This search will help you understand how you came to be You. Linking your values to your history will help you to bring them to mind more readily. In essence, this remembering helps you to see yourself more clearly and, when or if depression tries to make a comeback, you'll be ready with strongly rooted truths about who you are.

To begin, take one of the values or beliefs you uncovered and search your memory and history for other times when this value or belief was important. Do you have a memory of using this value? Can you remember acting on this belief? Did you adopt it from someone important to you? Did either of your parents or an important caregiver, grandparent, aunt, cousin, teacher or favourite story character ever model this value or belief?

Here is an example from my life:

I find that equality and fairness are important values in my life. They direct much of my action. They play out in my life through actions such as wanting to make sure that everyone has access to therapy, sharing my property and income with those that I care for, and being easily put off a conversation that smacks of sexism, racism, homophobia or gossip. When I discovered this about myself, I could easily see that my parents had helped create this part of my identity. I grew up with a pair of socialists on a hobby farm. We shared our labour with our neighbours and my parents often talked about left-leaning politics and the import- ance of unions. It wasn't until, years later, looking back at my high school graduation in 1982, that I understood just how these important values and beliefs were to me even as a youth.

When I reached forty and was contemplating the values of fairness and equality I had found, the memory from my gradu- ation day emerge. I clearly remembered the Valedictorian men- tioning my name and saying, "And Laurel Ewen (my maiden name) is likely to join the KKK and end racial prejudice forever".

Write down what comes to your mind. What is the story be- hind you coming to have your values or beliefs? There is a mem- ory or several memories for each of your values and beliefs. Take your time. Wait for these memories to arrive. Many people are pleasantly surprised by the memories that emerge.

The You, who you are now, was not born with an installed selection of values and beliefs. These identity markers were cre- ated, over time, in many contexts and through many important relationships. Your caregivers, peers, schools, neighbours, neigh- bourhoods, political ideas, conversations, media, social expect- ation and cultural messages moulded you. You were helped along to become who you are. You picked up some ideas and left other ideas behind. You chose to remember certain experiences and forget others. You actively went about, over time, adjusting and creating yourself.

The problem came about when you could not or did not live the life you created or wanted. The problem is here now to show you that you are not living according to what you want your life to be like – how you desire life to be, and that you are not achieving your ideal life because you are not adhering to your important values and beliefs. Remember, the problem is trying to make obvious that you are not living out the important values and beliefs that describe who you are. You made adjustments to yourself that resulted in the presence of depression. You did this for good reason. Survival!

Since birth, we have been taught that we need to act in ways that assure our survival. Unfortunately, some of these acts were contrary to important ways of life that you hold and, adhering to cultural ideas of safety that were meant to assure that you were never abandoned cause you to abandon your authentic self!

For each the five beliefs or five values you collected and wrote down, think of a story from the recent or distant past when you acted in accordance with them. For example, if one of your values is 'family', think of a time when you acted according to that value.

Collect five stories about a time (a minute, hour or day) when you acted in favour of what's important to you. You will be able to find these stories even if depression has been a part of life for many, many years. This is because you will still be acting in accordance with your values despite the presence of the problem. Journal these five points in time as small vignettes.

Now, look at each of these stories individually. Each story contains the steps you took to live life according to who you authentically are. Each story speaks of a time when you lived the way you wanted to despite the pressures of culture, society, family or friends to NOT be yourself. You will also have stories of living life despite the problem trying to stop you. And, you'll certainly have stories from before the problem got a good foothold in life.

These exceptions to the influence of the problem are moments (hours or even days) when you were YOU, AND the problem had no power. The problem has no power when YOU are being YOU! Remember, the problem is there to show you what you are NOT doing, that you SHOULD be doing. The problem got a foothold because you are or were NOT living according to your values and beliefs.

In each of these stories about life lived authentically, you will find you took certain steps to accomplish these moments or hours. These steps are better known as your skills and abilities. Your skills and abilities are acts that you use to accomplish a life lived according to what's important, according to your values. For example, I write to achieve fairness (value) and justice (value). A client of mine speaks up (value) for queer rights. Another client goes to meditation retreats to achieve awareness (value). My mother works with indigenous cultures, making sure their children have an education (value). My father builds and installs solar systems in small villages to bring lights to schools (education – value).

What do you do to bring your values to life? Write out some of the activities you enjoy doing and link these to the values or beliefs you discovered.

Once you have documented how (skills and abilities) you accomplished living according to what's important to you, in spite of the presence of the problem, narrow this information down to a few key sentences.

Example #1:
"I remember taking the kids to the park on a day when I would rather have stayed in bed. What I did to accomplish this was I let my love for the kids (passion, commitment . . .) be stronger than the depression. I just knew getting up and taking them was the right thing to do (integrity, virtuousness, good parenting, morality . . .)." The skill I used was to let my love for the kids be greater than the power of the problem.

Example #2:
When I was a kid I ran away from home often because my father was drunk all the time and he hit me. This memory came from thinking about a time when I used the value of justice in my life. I think I just wanted to be free (another value). The skill I used to do was determination. I was determined not to be hurt again.

Write a list of your skills and abilities. Make it as extensive as you like.

Next, using your imagination, think about what it would be like if, in the next few minutes, you used one or two of these skills and abilities to live your life despite the presence of depression; in accordance with what's important to you. How do you feel when you imagine this? What influence over life does depression have when you couple your skills and abilities to your values and beliefs? When you use your skills and abilities daily you're acting on your values. Acting according to your values and beliefs, through using your skills and abilities ensures that depression CANNOT get a foothold in life. The more you act according to your authentic self the less you need depression to point out that you are not being authentic. Depression becomes pointless.

How did you come to live with depression?

1. Depression came as a result of some missing, important beliefs, values, goals or dreams.

2. These important parts of life were suppressed by you. It is not your fault! Many factors led to you suppressing important ways of living. Not the least of which is your culture and social expectation. You changed to accommodate many ideas of what constitutes a "normal" life.

Changing who you were may have been the result of violence you experienced - either as a victim or onlooker. It might have been the result of acquiescing to cultural ideas about femininity or masculinity to achieve acceptance. Perhaps you were demeaned or humiliated in public and, to keep this from ever happening again, you changed yourself - hid yourself.

Living the life we imagined for ourselves takes the courage to make necessary changes. These changes are often opposite to the dictates – the wants and desires – of depression and the cultural conscripts set before us. It takes an immense amount of courage, faith and trust to turn our backs on the people who won't be supportive, and on ideas that do not work for us, but these changes are necessary in order to get back in touch with your authentic self.

Now that you know some values and beliefs, and skills and abilities that directly relate to who you are and what makes you unique, it is time to move your values and beliefs, through the use of your skills and abilities, into each new day. You are your authentic self when you are operating according to your values and beliefs.

Side Note: A few words about medication

If you're taking an antidepressant, please don't stop. Talk to your doctor about reducing the dose. Stopping an SSRI antidepressant (selective serotonin reuptake inhibitor) can result in a sudden decrease of serotonin levels throughout your body. Stopping could result in an increase in physical and/or psychological pain. If you're determined to stop, slowly withdraw under the direction of your doctor. As you practice living authentically, and as you withdraw from medication, monitor your thinking to see whether or not your brain has increased its own serotonin levels in sufficient amount to make you comfortable.

Bringing it all together

These are the therapeutic tasks you accomplished:

1. You named the problem.
2. You evaluated the influence this problem was having on your life.
3. You justified that influence by writing about whether or not you were OK with it.
4. You used the problem and its influence to find out what is important to you.
5. You did a lot of work to discover some values and beliefs that are very important to you.
6. You also traced the inception of these values and beliefs by looking at your history and some of the people and environment that played a role in their development.
7. You now know that your values, beliefs, commitments for living, goals and dreams speak about WHO YOU ARE.
8. You discovered the skills and abilities you have been successfully using against the influence of the problem, and that are linked to your values and beliefs.
9. Finally, you can be active in employing your skills and abilities to take control of the problem.

Leaving depression behind and moving into a new way of living life requires change. One cannot hold onto an old way of life AND have a different life at the same time. As you transition away from depression, don't be alarmed if a little chaos comes on the scene. Chaos is part of positive change. Sometimes it can feel as though the solid ground you were standing on has become like soft sand. It is shifting and moving in mysterious ways. That's ok. That is part of change.

"Transition is the natural process of disorientation and reorientation that marks the turning points in the path of growth . . . transitions are key times in the natural process of self-renewal"
William Bridges. Author of Managing Transitions: Making the Most of Change.

DIY RELIEF FROM CHRONIC PAIN

This therapy is one that is close to my heart. When I was completing my Master's degree at the University of Melbourne, Australia, I was asked to innovate a completely new therapeutic approach. Most of the other students directed their new therapies toward traditional problems such as depression, anxiety and so forth. I wanted to do something a bit more challenging so I decided to design a psychotherapy that dealt with chronic pain. At the time, I suffered greatly from osteoarthritis in my spine. I had had this problem for nearly 20 years. Often it was crippling and it caused me to see myself as the disabled one in my family. I had to ask for help when I wanted to stand up and, at night I had trouble walking to the bathroom. I had to quit many favoured activities, and I could no longer participate in many outdoor activities such as camping or kayaking.

During my Master's program, I put together a co-research team of people suffering in pain. The genesis of each participant's pain came from varying sources. There was a man with COPD (chronic obstructive pulmonary disease) who struggled to breathe, a woman with painful arthritic joints, another woman with neck injuries, a man with post-polio syndrome, and so on. Fifteen people in all participated. Together we applied a therapy

I designed to the problem of chronic, life-altering pain and we attempted to discover whether or not this new therapy altered pain in any significant way. The therapy was very successful.

When I presented our findings at the end of my Master's program, they were met with genuine, positive regard by students, teachers and therapist. Our therapy was taken on by a hospital team in China and was published in the 2016 edition of The International Journal of Narrative Therapy and Community Work.

The following DIY therapy has been constructed from some of that research and, since 2016 when I first designed this approach, I have added other effective techniques. Keep in mind, this approach to dealing with chronic pain is not meant to remove the problem that causes physiological pain. That's the domain of medicine. This therapy is about finding ways to sidestep the life-altering presence of physical pain and the resulting psychological distress. This DIY is about self-anaesthetic and strengthening ways of being and psychological wellness in the midst of chronic, traumatic or short-term pain. In short, it's about ways to live life that restore balance, reduce pain and reinstate identity lost to pain.

A Breakdown of this therapeutic process:
1. Uncover a strategy used against pain.
   Neil's story
   Pain takes us away from the knowledge of who we are
   Identifying what you love and have not lost to pain Your strategy
   The Synergistic Effect
2. Excavate the valued ways of living within this strategy
   Rest
   Recap
3. Allowing your strategy to expand into new ter tory.

Uncover a strategy used against pain

We all have times when pain is not towering over life. You may only be able to measure these times in seconds, but, for some people, these pain-relieved times can last hours. Something remarkably simple is happening during these pain-free moments. It is likely that, as you read these words, pain has had to take a back seat. This is because most humans do very poorly at concentrating on two distinct things at once, especially if our focus is on interesting subjects. We are very capable of holding seven, plus or minus two, pieces of information in our minds at any one point in time, but we are simply not able to focus on two separate physiological actions at the same time. Think about it. Are you able to focus both on breathing and swallowing at the same time? How about reading and running? You might be able to develop the ability to read and run at the same time, but neither action will get your full attention. Likewise, if you are focused a program on the radio as you drive, you'll likely find that you can't remember driving from one point to another. This is a type of amnesia where you completely forget how you got home.

Take a moment to think about a time during the day when pain does not dominate your thought – when you are completely immersed in an activity or some sensory action. Maybe it happens when you are watching TV or ironing clothes. It could happen while you listen to music or are yelling at the kids. Maybe you passed a restaurant and smelled delicious food and, for a few seconds, you thought about pulling over and eating.

Write that moment down. If you can remember other moments, write them down also. You might want to keep a piece of paper and pencil close and just document these moments over the next few hours. We are going to investigate what is happening during this time of being relatively pain-free.

Neil's story

Neil was part of our co-research team during my Master's program. At 65, one year after he was newly married to Mary, and shortly after they had both retired, they were both holiday diving off the coast of Mexico. Neil was a very experienced diver and he was endeavouring to teach Mary the ropes. The dive was not unusual in any degree. They were only 30 feet down, but when Neil came up he had developed Decompression Sickness 2 (DS2), a rare form of the diving phenomenon otherwise known as the bends. Shortly after Neil boarded the dive boat, his legs gave out from underneath him and he began vomiting. He went back to his palapa where they were staying but wasn't there for long before the dive instructor came to insist on Neil going to a nearby decompression chamber.

The decompression chamber would simulate the pressure of being under the water, which would reduce the size of the nitrogen bubbles that were now travelling up Neil's spine and cutting off the blood supply to his nerves. Neil was to stay in the decompression chamber until the nitrogen could be dissolved into his bloodstream, but by the time the dive instructor and Neil got going, the damage to his nervous system was beyond repair. To add to this, they encountered an accident on the highway that prevented them from getting to help for quite some time. This delay gave more opportunity to the damage being done to his spinal cord.

Neil spent a month in a Mexican hospital and two more months in a Canadian hospital back home. He spent the next two years in physiotherapy, pool therapy, trying acupuncture and chiropractic care, in a pain clinic and trying spinal blocks. He took Cymbalta, Lyrica, used fentanyl patches, marijuana pills (Sincimat) and a couple of joints. He tried Topiramate, but it gave him kidney stones. He tried different morphine strengths and time-release morphine, Lidocaine and ketamine infusions.

He tried a spinal cord stimulator, but the internal leads infected under his skin and had to be removed in an emergency. Nothing helped and there were several points in time when Neil thought to end the pain by taking his own life.

Pain takes us away from the knowledge of who we are

Neil and I spent hours investigating how pain had negatively influenced his life. He told me about all the things he couldn't do anymore. During our investigations, it was becoming evident that pain had a certain way of getting him to focus on what he had lost. I thought it might also be important to help Neil remember what pain had not managed to take from him. This, I thought, might act as an antidote to the depression that he suffered on account of the degree of loss he perceived. He had lost the ability to carry on in the direction of a big, important retirement dream he and Mary had. We didn't just step past the loss though. Instead, we acknowledged it and documented it. I intended to use it.

Lost dreams and lost activities due to chronic pain can be tremendously saddening because they often relate to a loss of identity, but that can also be used to point in the direction of important ways of living that need to be acknowledged and nourished – ways of life attached to values and beliefs that pain has undermined or diminished, but that are critical for the maintenance of hope and equally important to the development of new dreams.

Take some time out to make a list of what pain has taken from you. Allow yourself to mourn the loss of these things; of the dreams and hopes you had for the future that have been cut short by pain. Think of the activities you can no longer take part in. Be saddened by this loss. These are things that you will be leaving behind as we progress forward. Leaving them behind will likely create the sense that there is a hole in life, but I intend for you to fill this hole with newness – with new activities and a renewed, and perhaps clearer, sense of who you are.

When I made my list, and when Neil and other researchers made their lists, we noticed that what we had lost spoke of what we valued. What we had lost pointed to the goals and dreams we had been harbouring for years - some of which came to fruition and others that were still waiting for us to accomplish, but that would now never see the light of day. These lost activities seemed to speak of who we were and losing them also told us that we were losing a significant part of ourselves.

In a certain way, these thoughts and feelings about the loss of hopes and dreams and the accompanying feeling that you have lost a great part of yourself are true, but it doesn't capture the whole picture of life. Our job is going to be finding other symbols, similar to the ones lost through pain and disability, that will replace the lost ones, but that hold the same, if not greater, significance. These symbols will coincide with what you value, but will also be used to create activities that can numb pain, renew hope and strengthen identity. In turn, a stronger identity will undermine pain and loss and open new direction in life, despite pain.

Identifying what you love and have not lost to pain

Previously, you hopefully were able to make a pretty detailed (and maybe somewhat painful) list of things that pain has taken from you. Neil's list included some of the following:

I can't work on cars.

I can't dive.

I can't travel.

I can't walk for very long or any great distance.

All I can do is sit with my feet up, pet the dog and watch TV.

We began to investigate what this loss meant about what was important to him. I asked Neil what he watched on TV. Not surprisingly, he watched travel documentaries, car and DIY programs. I asked him what pain was doing while he participated in these acts? What he noticed was that during these programs he was, off and on, pain-free. He had inadvertently found a way to distract himself from the influence of pain, but he hadn't made the connection between doing something he liked and the absence of pain. He had not given much thought to how effective watching a favourite TV program had been against pain until this fact was made visible through our research. These distractions were of great interest to him and we began to think of using them more deliberately.

Instead of thinking, "All I can do is sit with my feet up, pet the dog and watch TV", he could now think, "To relieve myself of pain, I could sit and watch a DIY program or a travel documentary". The depth of interest in these programs made watching TV a great pain reliever, but it would also be important to investigate why he loved these programs - what values and beliefs were attached to this strategy and how could we use those values and beliefs to uncover more strategies against pain?

Neil could still drive and he discovered that this was the greatest pain reliever of all. While driving, Neil could not be distracted by pain. He was concerned with safety and concentrating on the road, on driving. If anything did distract him it was the sight of a car he greatly admired. This act - driving - was reintroduced into Neil's life as a strategy he could use against pain. This strategy fit with what he believed was important, namely, travelling and cars. By highlighting what he was doing to reduce his pain, and some things could still do, we were making him more conscious of his power over pain. We learned that Neil had not lost everything dear to him to pain. He was still able to travel in his motorhome. He was still able to enjoy mechanics by watching DIY programs. And, although he would never dive again, he used his knowledge to warn other divers of the possibility of injury.

Your strategy

When are you the most distracted? Is it when you are cooking, reading, texting, surfing on the web, talking on the phone, driving? Pay attention throughout the day to when pain has little or no influence on life. You will find that these times are filled with activities that you most enjoy and that are highly distracting. For example, as I write this therapy out for publishing, I have no evidence of pain in my body. I can stop and think about the pain and experience it, but as soon as I return to typing and thinking again, the pain is absent. This is because I love to write and think. These two activities fit with important ways of living life namely, helping others and creating. The coupling of these two values (helping and creating) to their accompanying activities (writing and thinking) is similar to a one-two punch – a double dose of analgesic.

Have a note pad handy and write down the times when pain is not available. Write down what you are doing. For example, Pain is not available when I am knitting. Pain is not available when I am working. Pain is not available when I am walking the dog, listening to a podcast, watching a travel program (food program, building program, design, and beauty. . .) on TV, talking on the phone, surfing the web . . .

Now, take some time to re-read what you have written and to think about each of these activities. What about these activities is enjoyable for you? Is it that you have always enjoyed feeding others, or eating good food? Is it that you think helping others is important? What is it? The 'what' we are looking for will equate to the values and beliefs you hold dear and precious. These values and beliefs are easy for you to act upon because they are part of who you are. They are your identity markers.

Here is another example.

Earl was also part of our research study. He suffered daily

with chronic pain and COPD. Often, despite the pain, he would take daily rides around the neighbourhood on his golf cart with his two beloved dogs. During these rides, he was not thinking about pain. When we investigated what was happening while he was out and about, we discovered that Earl was engaging in many visits and conversations and he was taking the dogs out to pee and to see things. We looked into what these activities meant in terms of what Earl valued and we learned that he valued connections (value) with friends and caring (value) about his pets. As long as Earl was able to connect with friends and care about his pets pain could not dominate his life. Similarly, if Earl had friends over for conversation, he was relatively pain-free.

Earl's activity of driving around in his golf cart was re-termed as a strategy he used against pain. Along with this re-terming, I made it evident that this activity connected to his values of caring and connecting. We also took time to investigate the genesis of these values by asking Earl how long he had held them, how he might have come to adopt them and in what other areas of life could he see these values at work? Together we traced these values back many years.

The Synergistic Effect

No two people will discover the same effective strategy for combating pain because people are created in specific, unique environments and in concert with significant people over years of existence. Also, added to this is the process of remembering and forgetting. People choose which experiences to remember and which to forget. And, alongside or intermingled with both of the above factors, and contributing to uniqueness, is each person's hierarchical placement of their beliefs and values. One person might believe justice is the most important value to hold and would, therefore, place this value at the top of all other values they hold. Another might think justice is important, but not the most important value to hold and so place it beneath other values of greater importance. We all have a hierarchy of values - the placement and use of values as we make decisions in life. No two people will think or act exactly the same because of the outside influencing factors that help to shape the valued they hold and in which order in a hierarchy they hold them. What people do have in common, however, is the result of less pain when they employ a strategy that is rooted in values and beliefs they hold dear. And, if an effective strategy is uncovered, the results can be synergistic.

Not only do people find that when they employ an effective strategy that they are not thinking about the pain and have achieved an analgesic effect, but while they are enjoying actions that quiet pain and that arise from the strategy, they are able to produce more health and quicker recovery times. When people engage in acts that arise from their personalized strategy or strategies, the outcome of those acts is not more pain, but less, even if they are doing activities that generally would increase pain had they not been in accordance with valued ways of living. Added to this effect is the result of living more authentically. Using strategies that are grounded in important valued and beliefs bring people closer to who they are. Values and beliefs are identity markers and, when these are actively practised, the effect is a stronger knowledge of self.

For example, a client decided that her strategy was to get out for hikes in the forest. She had been suffering from chronic back pain for eighteen years. This was the result of degenerating disks in both her upper and lower spine. X-rays and CAT scans had confirmed that the disks were beginning to crumble and press together. Soon she would begin to feel pain in her legs that indicated that her nerves were being compressed and cut off. Her doctor told her that there was no cure and he informed her that, eventually, she would have to undergo back surgery. Back surgery has a notorious history of going wrong and this was not something that she wanted.

She loved the outdoors, especially gardening and the ocean. Chronic pain had taken many outdoor activities from her, such as kayaking and landscaping, and she was resolved to sit for hours in her easy chair with nothing to do but watch TV and knit. As we talked about uncovering an effective strategy, she thought that going outdoors would help if it didn't cause more pain, which usually it did. Because she had a dog that needed daily walks, she started trying out a strategy of walking. She learned about some local trails and began walking some local paths. Within days of her commitment to walk, her eldest son came to her and asked she would like to go on a hike with him. He was an avid hiker. She did go and they went on a fairly strenuous, two-kilometre hike uphill and back down. At the end of it, she was tired, but surprisingly she felt no pain, neither on the hike nor after. She knew then, that she had found the action associated with her strategy that would work for her.

When we looked at the values and beliefs that were associated with this activity, we found out about the importance of staying fit and being healthy. Her father was eighty two and he was still fit, healthy and able to enjoy many outdoor activities. She was resolved to carry on as her father had.

This client is now hiking over nine kilometres twice a week. Her back pain is less because the muscles in her hips, and torso have increased. This muscle increase has helped protect the degenerating disks and has stabilized her back, allowing her to participate in many activities that before had resulted in debilitating pain. On top of this, she has reported having wonderful meditative experiences while in the forest, not suffering guilt from neglecting the dog and having better sleep at night. If she were to find another strategy that encompassed her valued ways of living - staying fit and healthy - she would then have two ways of quieting pain.

Excavate the valued ways of living within this strategy

Once you know what strategy you use to distract yourself from pain, the next step is to investigate why this is so effective. The effectiveness will be found in the values and beliefs that drive the strategy. I have given a couple examples above, but here are some questions to help you uncover what your strategy is and what it says about what's important to you. This information will help you get to the next step of strengthening identity that may have been undermined by pain. You'll accomplish this by moving your values and beliefs into other activities/strategies.

Complete the following statements in your notebook or on a piece of paper.

1. I am most distracted from pain when I am _____ (fill in the activity that distracts you the most). Try to get two or more activities written down.

2. I am enjoying this activity because I believe _____ (helping others, being outdoors, cooking. . . whatever you wrote in statement 2) is an important part of life or way of living.

3. I learned this way of life from _____ (mother, father, aunt, favourite character. . .).

4. I am enjoying this activity because it fit with the values of _____ that I hold dear.

Remember to check the list of values in the appendix if you need help identifying these important ways of living and being.

Try to gather three or more values or beliefs. Below is a framework for writing out your strategy, the values that make it effective and the origin of this way of life. This example is from my life.

I am distracted from pain when I am in therapy sessions with others. I am enjoying this activity because I believe that helping (value) others is important. My mother and father taught me this. I grew up among socialists and learned very early in life the importance of sharing (value) time and helping others. I help others by giving (value) away my time, sharing my income, writing books and studying to improve (believe statement that could reduce 'advance') to my therapeutic skills. I enjoy these activities because they fit with other values of fairness, giving, creating and supporting others and my family.

For each activity you wrote down, write out something similar to my statement above.

Rest

In the above work, you did a lot of thinking. I suggest you take a break, close this book and spend some time doing something else. This rest will help you integrate the material you've learned. It will also give the opportunity for new ideas and strategies to emerge.

Recap

People are most distracted from pain when they are engaging in activities that connect with values, beliefs and commitments for living that are important to them. This is because when we are engaging in value-based or belief-based activities we are being true to ourselves - we are being authentic. Authenticity is a cornerstone of an effective strategy. This type of activity is most distracting because, being ourselves, or being authentic, is the most rewarding way of living life. Have you ever had the experience of going to a professional about pain just to have them send you home with exercises to do or mindfulness to practice? You probably went home and tried these practices for a few days, but soon became bored and gave up. The reason for this is that neither of these acts (exercise or meditation) fits with your valued ways of living. They are poor strategies.

Pain would have us believe that we cannot do the things we love and that we have suffered more loss than we could ever gain back. This, in turn, causes us to think that we cannot be the person we want to be, or that the person we were has been lost forever. This thinking leads to thoughts of loss and sadness. Sadness and loss lead to depression and, sometimes, depression can lead to suicide. In truth, we cannot do some things that we used to do, but we can still do many things that reflect what we value and believe. There are a lot of activities we have yet to be introduced to. Most times, these new activities are just as rewarding as the ones we left behind. To access them, you will need to be patient and remain open to the possibilities that lie outside your current view of the world.

Take some time to sit quietly and open your mind to the myriad of possibilities that lie just outside your current consciousness. You might be very surprised about what comes your way.

Allowing your strategy to expand into new territory

It is important that, once you have found your specific way of quieting pain in life, you allow this strategy to expand into other areas of life. For example if, like Terry, you find that being outdoors is effective, check out different outdoor spaces to determine which one is desirable and most effective. You will have an established repertoire of activities that you're holding in your thinking, but these acts are not the only ones that can be implemented. You might not have thought of many other actions that will have an even more profound effect on pain.

To allow your strategy to expand, you will have to let go of KNOWING. What this means is that you need to take to heart the FACT that you don't know all the actions associated with your strategy and, if you only use those acts that you know about, you'll be missing out on the ones that are likely to be the most effective or enjoyable. The most effective acts will come to you from unexpected places or people and in "common hours" (re-

read the opening quote at the beginning of this book by Thoreau). Stay open to this and you'll discover the BEST way to be with your strategy. In the beginning, use what you have, but stay open and in a welcoming state of mind as you carry on. Remember, your strategy is wrapped around your values and beliefs, and the act or acts that arise from these will have compounding or synergistic effects on your physiological AND psychological self. I've listed some of these effects below.

Physiological effects:
Stronger body
Healthier body
Less pain or no pain
Healing or diminished recovery time

Psychological effects:
Better mental health (less anger or depression)
A sense of belonging, happiness, and/or a positive sense of direction
More positive brain chemistry (endorphins, dopamine, norepinephrine, and serotonin)
Less anxiety or worry about the future
A greater sense of authenticity

These don't happen all at once but are rather an effect of practising your strategic actions against pain. Pain is not a natural or welcome part of any life and so, working to make positive pain-alterations have the effect of altering many other areas of life for the better. This is your body and brain working with you to achieve homeostasis. In a way, you are using pain to uncover a more authentic or natural way of living.

Remember, strategies that fit with what you value and belief also fit with who you are because your values and beliefs are your identity markers. A strategy against pain that is effective will increase your desire for and enjoyment of life. Your strategy or strategies against pain will have the effect of improving life each

Laurel A. Phillips

time you use it.

DIY RELIEF FROM OBSESSIVE THOUGHT: DEPRESSION, ANGER AND NEGATIVE RUMINATION

This DIY therapy is used to combat thinking that leads to negative and paralyzing rumination and that can result in depression, anger, suicidal ideation, aggressive behaviour, frustration, disappointment or a profound sense of being lost. If you are struggling with runaway, out-of-control thinking then this DIY is for you.

A breakdown of this therapeutic process:
1. Catching negative thinking in motion.
   Thoughts are energy.
   Energy leads to action
2. Identifying the original negative thought (N)
   Noticing
   Digging back

3. Negative thinking (NN) about the original neg
tive thought
   The purpose of N
   Overwhelming
   Recap
   Ego
   Recap
4. Putting a stop to the original negative thought (N)
   Recap
5. Healing
   Using N to gain insight

Catching negative thinking in motion

This first step is not very difficult to do, but it is crucial for a very important reason. In catching yourself thinking negatively or ruminating (the phrase psychologist use for continuous and repetitive negative thinking), you remove yourself from being someone for whom negative thinking is simply happening to, to being someone who watches her or his negative thinking happening. The difference is subtle but important. Once you notice that you are thinking negative thoughts you're in the position to have this insight: I am not my thought. I am the person observing my thought. I am the generator of thoughts. I can stop my thought by not generating it.

Thoughts are Energy

If you take an object such as a chair or table and you look at it under an electron microscope you'll see that it is made up of atoms. If you then take an atom from that object and break it apart (you'll need a particle accelerator), and then take the particles of that busted atom and break them apart, and you continue to do this to the protons and electrons until there is nothing left to break apart, you'll find that you are left with only energy. Everything is made of energy. This energy is brought together in certain atomic combinations such as a table, chair, bed, tree, animal or human. The earth and all matter, plus everything between points of matter, is just waves of energy. This is important to know because your thoughts are not solid objects. They are not solid masses of things in your head. They are just waves of energy moving in and out of your mind. They are bits of energy, coming together for moments and then slipping apart.

Thoughts are often accompanied by images produced in your imagination. Imagination is our ability to shape thoughts into pictures. Imagination uses energy to generate emotion and emotion is used to generate more thought. Imagination, emotion, and thought form a type of thinking feedback loop. This loop or process is meant to generate more energy. The reason for this energy generation is, in the end, to produce an action.

Energy Leads to Action

All thought, both negative and positive, is energy in motion. Thoughts are about yourself and your life and, in the case of obsessive thinking, can lead to a compounding of negative and catastrophic thinking about the past, present or future. Desires to end your life, medicate yourself, distract yourself, engage in unhealthy activities or lash out at yourself and others are the result of runaway, negative thinking. Runaway thought can be about the actions of others, either real or imagined. This leads to blaming, hating, withdrawal, lashing out against others, running away from relationships, jobs or other relational connections.

You are the generator of your thoughts, both negative and positive. You therefore are the generator of thought energy for the purpose of carrying out an act or action. All thought, as energy, is meant to produce an energetic result or an ACTION. For most people, this need to act or produce action is unconscious. The thought of wanting something does not typically begin with the thought of wanting it. For example, when you want a choc-olate bar, this want seems begins with a driving desire for some-thing sweet, and not with a thought of 'chocolate bar'. Most people don't know about the thought that underlies the desire. Most are only aware of the need to have chocolate. The need or desire is emotion birthed from an initial, unconscious thought.

The thought of wanting something (or not wanting or doing or not doing), and the act that is generated to get it, is undergirded by an original thought, but for most of us, the initial thought is not obvious. Most only recognize the emotion that has surfaced from the unrecognized, unconscious, initial thought. The initial thought, bred an emotion (desire, in the case of the chocolate) and then, from the emotion of desire, we have another thought, "I want a chocolate bar". For most of us, the process of action seems to be this: want = thinking = action.

A thought, however, is preceding the step before emotion (ex. desire). Emotions are the step before action. You have an initial, unconscious thought that creates an emotion that then creates another thought that then breeds action. That initial, uncon-scious thought is very small and can go unnoticed. It begins as a small point of energy. On top of this small point of energy is placed a bit more energy in the form of an emotion. This then generates more energy in the form of more thought. Added to the initial point of energy (the unconscious thought) is emotional energy and more thought energy and more emotional energy, all piled on top of that original pinprick of energy.

Runaway thinking is the process of adding more energy and more thoughts and more emotions to an initial unconscious thought. This is the production of rumination. Rumination is like pouring gasoline on a thought fire. It creates serious amounts of emotional energy and can easily become an almost unstop-pable thinking process. If this process is maintained, a person will think that the only way to end this horrible, powerful, think-ing-cycle of negative rumination is to ACT. NOW! If, however, an action is delayed, for whatever reason, a type of paralysis can set in. People tend to fold in on themselves when this happens.

This folding in can manifest in taking substances, daylong TV watching, hiding out at home, or other solo activities meant to distract from the energy overload. Staying put and succumbing to thoughts and emotion can culminate in ideas of suicide as the only way out.

The beginning motivation to this whole process of negative rumination still remains outside of awareness, in the subconscious, and is the original thought that began the entire negative thinking process.

Recap

You are not your thought.

You are the generator of thoughts.

You can observe your thoughts.

Thoughts are not solid things. They are energy. Their reality is as an energy wave and not a solid thing.

Imagination and emotion use energy to generate more thinking.

Energy needs a release. That release is an action. You want this action and so you create a way to get this action to happen. That 'way' is through creating energy in the form of an initial thought. This initial thought comes from your subconscious. It is not conscious to you. It is not in your field of awareness.

Identifying the original negative thought

Although many of the steps that lead up to rumination and acting out in negative ways can be recognized, one step in this process takes uncovering. This step is the recognition of the original negative thought (N). By the time most people get to the point of fight or flight (the action birthed from negative rumination), lots of thinking has transpired. Most, if not all, of this thinking seems to be thrusting itself upon us, but as I wrote earlier, we are the generators of this thought onslaught. It just appears to be happening to us without our consent. An original negative thought (N) sparked this barrage of negative thinking.

The recognition of this N is where we need to get to, and where we are going next.

Noticing

Recognizing N is going to begin by your recognition of rumination. We'll start here, at rumination, because this is the point where most people are able to recognize that thinking is happening, and that it is out of control. At the high point of rumination, a person knows that thinking is harming them. This rumination is also known as negative thinking about the original negative thought or NN. YOU MUST CATCH YOURSELF BEING CAUGHT UP IN NN in order to trace back to N. When you recognize that you are caught up in NN, acknowledge this. Say to yourself, "I'm ruminating" or "I'm thinking negatively" or "I'm generating many negative thoughts right now". Step back and catch one or two of those thoughts. Look at them. Acknowledge them. Write them down. Remind yourself that these are bits of energy piled on top of other bits of energy, nothing more. These are all waves of energy, as all things are, formed into thoughts, piled one on top of each other and fueled by emotion, imagination and rumination.

These thoughts are energizing your imagination, which, in turn, is generating more energy and more emotion, and this is forming into more thoughts. You are doing this. You are moving this energy about. It may not feel like you are in control, but you are.

Digging Back

The only way to permanently cease this NN rumination is to trace your thoughts back to the N – the original negative thought. Here's how to do that:

1. Write down three or four of the NNs your hearing in your head.
2. These thoughts will have a common thread.
3. That common thread is FEAR.

4. Fear is part of the N you need to get to, but it is only part. The other part is what this fear is telling you.

5. Go back to your list of NNs. Add a few more if you can. Don't be afraid. Remember, its only energy, nothing more. This energy can't hurt you.

6. Try to decipher what the NNs are telling you to fear? What do they want you to run away from? Read your list of NNs and ask yourself, "What are these telling me to fear?"

Here is n example.

Evelyn wants to leave her husband (an action). Once every few months she feels herself hating him (NN). The whole hating episode starts with thoughts of not trusting him (NN), disliking him (NN), loathing him (NN). Eventually, she gets to the point of ruminating for a few hours, eventually withdrawing her love (an action) and making plans to leave him (an action).

She decides to investigate the most recent episode of this recycling phenomenon. She looks back as far as she can and tries to recall the beginning f the experience. She recalls being with her husband in the kitchen and telling him about something exciting that had happened that day. She remembers thinking that he seemed not to care (NN).

Evelyn wrote down this NN and others that came.

He doesn't care about me
He's being unfaithful.
He's going to hurt me one day.
He's hiding something.

When she investigated these ruminating thoughts for a common thought associated with FEAR, she realized that she was afraid that he was trying to hurt her (N). She wrote this FEAR down.

Fear of being hurt.

What prompted the NN barrage that lead Evelyn to make plans to leave her husband was a FEAR of being hurt. FEAR of being hurt is Evelyn's N – her original thought.

Evelyn wondered why she might hold this fear in her subconscious. Taking time to look at her history, she saw that many men had harmed her in the past and that she was always afraid of it happening again. She had been beaten several times by three different men. This abuse began with her father when she was a little girl. She had been raped twice as an adult by men she trusted. She had been demeaned, put down, mind-gamed and made to feel insignificant and ugly by men.

Once you have put a label on what your ruminating thoughts are trying to tell you – of what 'fear' is generating them - then it becomes easy to identify the N of your subconscious thinking.

Negative thinking about the original negative thought

In Evelyn's case (a true story), the N was Fear of being hurt. It had to be uncovered using the NNs of rumination because it was outside of her awareness. When her husband came home, she didn't think, "I'm afraid he is going to hurt me!" What she felt was the emotion of anger. This anger came through an interpretation of his behaviour. Evelyn's N was using her husband to generate energy. The emotion of anger was two, or perhaps even three degrees away from N and still. Evelyn was so far removed from the recognition of her own thinking, of N, that she blamed her husband for how she was thinking and feeling. At this great distance from N, she began to trace back through the many emotions and NNs. The NNs lead her to N.

The NN's will also lead you to your N. Don't worry if you're uncertain as to whether or not you can perfectly articulate your N. Your N is going to be fear-based. All Ns are. All you need to uncover is a response to the question, 'FEAR of what?'

The purpose of N

All NNs are generated, by you, from an N. That is the purpose of N – to have you gather energy by generating many NNs. NNs serve to justify the original negative thought (N), to keep it safe and alive. Why? Because this N is such a huge part of who you think you are. The original negative thought (N) is the ground on which your negative thought about who you think you are is kept alive. You keep N alive to justify who you think you are. You might do this to the point of exhaustion. The N is draining all your energy. This N is also working hard to maintain an illusion. You are keeping this illusion of who you are alive by keeping N safe through feeding it the energy of NNs and emotions and imagination.

That's a lot to take in. If you need to, read it again until it sinks in.

Overwhelming

Remember that N arrives unannounced. It is living in your subconscious. You buried it there. It is energy – pure, unadulterated energy. I'll explain that later. N is not the problem. N has been generated from a negative incident or experience in your past. N is the energy produced from a past, negative experience and it is the sign that some identity-altering has occurred. You can use N, once you have uncovered it and brought it into awareness, to find the identity-altering incident. Once that has been pulled from subconsciousness, you will be able to dismiss it and reunite with your authentic self. You have some work to do first.

Recap

NNs are food for N.
NNs generate a lot of additional energy.
Without an avenue for escape, this energy can be overwhelming.

It can also be paralyzing.

NNs have the ability to narrow your thinking. After ruminating for an hour, a day, or even a week or two, you will find that thoughts of other things have been squeezed out. Action has been stopped.

Everything, all thought energy and energy from elsewhere in your body is now in service to feeding the N. This is done in order to keep the N alive.

Keeping the N alive is done so you can keep this idea of yourself alive. This idea of you is part of the illusion of who you think you are, but not who you really are and it was generated through a significant, negative, past experience.

Ego

NNs are conceptual. This means that NNs generate concepts about who you are. These concepts are akin to little slices of N. They and the original negative thought (N) are also in service to keeping an idea of separateness alive. This separateness is the isolating effect of the illusion of identity that the harmful past experience brought about. All humans maintain an idea of who they are, but this idea is not always helpful.

Separateness comes from the idea that we are unique and not like anyone else. This sense of separateness is also termed ego. Your ego is the culmination of ideas about yourself and it is chiefly concerned with separating you out from others as special, even if that specialness is grounded in pain. Ego is constructed through all the ideas you have about yourself, whether true or not, picked up throughout your lifetime. N is part of your ego

When you uncover the N and, are subsequently able to see the painful, past incident on which N is founded, you'll have the opportunity to remove this original thought from your identity. You'll be able to stop N from generating any more energy through your observance of N and the recognition that N is only a pinpoint of energy. When N no longer has the power to generate energy and keep itself alive, it is removed from your ego-idea library. It can then no longer participate in the constitution of your identity. When this happens, you'll experience an ego shift. This shift will be away from who you thought you were toward who you authentically are. This shift might feel somewhat unsettling at first because you're moving away from the ground of your illusion, all that was in place to maintain that illusion, to a more solid ground of reality. Allow the shakiness to happen. Remind yourself that it is a normal part of becoming who you truly are.

Recap

You can find your N by looking at your NNs.

N is fear-based.

N needs energy to survive. NNs are feeding it and keeping it alive.

N is kept alive so that an idea/illusion of who you are can
be kept alive.

NNs are about concepts of SELF or, ideas about who one
is. They are small slices of N.

Ego is your idea of who you are. This idea causes
separateness and feelings of being unique or different from everyone else – even if that uniqueness is grounded in pain.

Ego is an illusion. Moreover, if the illusion of who you are is founded in a painful and harmful experience and is allowed to remain alive there is little room for authenticity to emerge.

Putting a stop to the original negative thought

This is not as hard as you might think. Once you have traced NNs to N, stopping N from influencing life is done through observation. N is only energy, but it is not like the energy of NNs. NNs are impure energy. N is pure energy. NNs are created by you and are completely negative (when we are talking about rumination and negative thinking). They are created in service to feeding N. N is pure energy. It is neither good nor bad. It just is. N came on the scene of your life through a harmful experience. This experience altered your concept of self and generated an illusory identity. The experience took you away from who you really are - away from your authenticity. This DIY is about moving you back into a state of authenticity.

For the sake of uncovering N, we labelled it FEAR and we expanded this definition with Fear of . . . (whatever you uncovered through looking at your NNs). In reality, this energy, pure energy - is neither positive nor negative. I had you attach a label to it in order for you to more easily recognize it. For this next step in the process, I want you to peel that label off. You can use the label to help you continue to recognize N in the future and stop NNs, but for right now, take the label off. We can use Evelyn's N and her process as an example. Fear of being hurt.

Evelyn peeled back all the NNs to look at her N. She then peeled off the label of 'Fear of being hurt' and gave it a more appropriate label, 'Energy'. That's what it was, pure energy. She then removed any associated qualities attached to this energy. N, the original point of energy, was neither good or bad. It became, in her mind's eye, just a wave of energy, because that's all it really was. When the N is seen for what it truly is, just energy without any ideas, concepts, qualities or identifiers attached, it cannot have you generate NNs. If you cannot generate NNs, the N gets no extra energy. No energy = no life.

Try this now.

Close your eyes and see your FEAR as a point of energy. You can imagine this point as though it is a small pinprick of light.
Remove the label of 'Fear' from it.
Wipe away any quality of good or bad.
The pinprick of energy is from your past, negative experience.
Notice that this small light is not generating any thought or emotion. It just is. It is there.

Recap
Once you have labelled the N, then you can peel the label off and

identify it as pure energy. That's all it is, energy.

This energy is neither good nor bad. It needs no qualities or ideas attached to it. It need only be recognized as energy.

Seen for what it is, N is unable to cause us to generate NNs.

No NNs means no food for N. No food for N = the end the influence of N on thinking.

When rumination is recognized, go to the source.

Remember N and see it as simple, pure energy. NNs will fall like a house of cards in the wind.

Healing

I've given you steps to end not only the barrage of thought that leads to depression, anger, paralysis, fear, and a host of flight or fight acts, but I have also brought you to a point of potential healing. This healing involves insight.

Insight, as I am using the term, means the heartfelt knowledge of who one truly is. This is the knowledge that brings healing. Insight is an epiphany. It is not generated through your thinking, but rather, it is a new knowledge that comes from the source of everything. It is universal knowledge and it cannot be generated from scholarly study or from a downloading of information. Insight emerges from a place deep with each of us, but its source is not individual. Rather, the source of insight is the collective consciousness - the source of all knowledge that we can all tap into but that no individual can lay claim to. Insight is not learned and it cannot be bought. It is akin to a gift from the universe, or God or whatever you believe is the source of all things seen and unseen. Insight is registered as capital 'T' truth. It is not conceptual knowledge and, therefore, does not cause separateness as ego does. Insight knowledge brings healing and compassion for both the individual and for others. This DIY therapy has been generated from insight knowledge. Knowledge and compassion brought by insight knowledge are extended simultaneously to self and others.

Using N to gain insight

When you are able to see N as simple, unlabeled energy, the pain that produced N is unveiled. For Evelyn, she understood that FEAR of being hurt was generated by being seriously harmed throughout her life by several men. Through seeing N as simple energy, she was able to let go of this pain and the idea that it could happen again. She was set free from this fear and this, in turn, left a space in her life to be filled with healing and compassion. She could now see and understand that the people who hurt her were hurting themselves and that they had been hurt badly in their lives. She felt empathy for them. She could acknowledge that she was ready to hurt her husband, to leave him, to withdraw her love from him because of this hurt. She now understood that withdrawing love and leaving were only acts that perpetuated the pain she was feeling and guaranteed her more pain and/or that she would continue to pass on the pain, like a virus, to other partners. She had gained insight knowledge and true understanding. She had used her pain to heal herself. That was the purpose of N, to help Evelyn heal.

Remember to take time to let this healing sink in and take shape in life. Making room for something new by ending an outmoded way of existing can often leave people feeling a bit empty. Don't concern yourself with this feeling, if it comes your way. Soon, the space you made will fill with a new reality and insight. Take time to welcome this healing into life.

APPENDIX

List of Values

This is a very extensive list of values. If you are resorting to searching for an appropriate value by going over this list, do yourself the favour of trusting your intuition. Take a few moments to reassure yourself that what is important to you, the values you hold, are here. As you read through the list, let those important values emerge, rather than sweat about which you should pick. Let the values pick you. Write down the ones that stand out for you or that. When you have a list, look at it, read it over and try to condense it to four or five. You'll find that many you've picked have a similar meaning.

Abundance Acceptance Accessibility Accomplishment Accountability Accuracy Achievement Acknowledgement Activeness Adaptability Adoration Adroitness Advancement Adventure Affection Affluence Aggressiveness Agility Alertness Altruism Amazement Ambition Amusement Anticipation Appreciation Approachability Approval Art Articulacy Artistry Assertiveness Assurance Attentiveness Attractiveness Audacity Availability Awareness Awe Balance Beauty Being the best Belonging Benevolence Bliss Boldness Bravery Brilliance Buoyancy Calmness Camaraderie Candor Capability Care Carefulness Celebrity Certainty Challenge Change Charity Charm Chastity Cheerfulness Clarity Cleanliness Clear-mindedness Cleverness Closeness Comfort Commitment Community Compassion Competence Competition Completion Composure Concentration Confidence Conformity Congruency Connection   Consciousness Conservation Consistency Contentment Continuity Contribution Control Conviction Conviviality Coolness Cooperation Cordiality Correctness Country Courage Courtesy Craftiness Creativity Credibility Cunning Curiosity Daring Decisiveness Decorum Deference Delight Dependability Depth Desire Determination Devotion Devoutness Dexterity Dignity Diligence Direction Directness Discipline Discovery Discretion Diversity Dominance Dreaming Drive Duty Dynamism Eagerness Ease Economy Ecstasy Education Effectiveness Efficiency Elation Elegance Empathy Encouragement Endurance Energy Enjoyment Entertainment Enthusiasm Environmentalism Ethics Euphoria Excellence Excitement Exhilaration Expectancy Expediency Experience Expertise Exploration Expressiveness Extravagance Extroversion Exuberance Fairness Faith Fame Family Fascination Fashion Fearlessness Ferocity Fidelity Fierceness Financial- independence Firmness Fitness Flexibility Flow Fluency Focus Fortitude Frankness Freedom Friendliness Friendship Frugality Fun Gallantry Generosity Gentility Giving Grace Gratitude Gregariousness Growth Guidance Happiness Harmony Health Heart Helpfulness Heroism Holiness Honesty Honor Hopefulness Hospitality Humility Humor Hygiene Imagination Impact Impartiality Independence Individuality Industry Influence Ingenuity Inquisitiveness Insightfulness Inspiration Integrity Intellect Intelligence Intensity Intimacy Intrepidness Introspection Introversion Intuition Intuitiveness Inventiveness Investing Involvement Joy Judiciousness Justice Keenness Kindness Knowledge Leadership Learning Liberation Liberty Lightness Liveliness Logic Longevity Love Loyalty Majesty Making a difference Marriage Mastery Maturity Meaning Meekness Mellowness Meticulousness Mindfulness Modesty Motivation Mysteriousness Nature Neatness Nerve Noncomformity Obedience Open-mindedness Openness Optimism Order Organization Originality Outdoors Outlandishness Outrageousness Partnership Patience Passion Peace Perceptiveness Perfection Perkiness Perseverance Persistence Persuasiveness Philanthropy Piety Playfulness Pleasantness Pleasure Poise Polish Popularity

Potency Power Practicality Pragmatism Precision Preparedness Presence Pride Privacy Proactivity Professionalism Prosperity Prudence Punctuality Purity Rationality Realism Reason Reasonableness Recognition Recreation Refinement Reflection Relaxation Reliability Relief Religiousness Reputation Resilience Resolution Resolve Resourcefulness Respect Responsibility Rest Restraint Reverence Richness Rigor Sacredness Sacrifice Sagacity Saintliness Sanguinity Satisfaction Science Security Self-control Selflessness Self-reliance Self-respect Sensitivity Sensuality Serenity Service Sexiness Sexuality Sharing Shrewdness Significance Silence Silliness Simplicity Sincerity Skillfulness Solidarity Solitude Sophistication Soundness Speed Spirit Spirituality Spontaneity Spunk Stability Status Stealth Stillness Strength Structure Success Support Supremacy Surprise Sympathy Synergy Teaching Teamwork Temperance Thankfulness Thoroughness Thoughtfulness Thrift Tidiness Timeliness Traditionalism Tranquility Transcendence Trust Trustworthiness Truth Understanding Unflappability Uniqueness Unity Usefulness Utility Valor Variety Victory Vigor Virtue Vision Vitality Vivacity Volunteering Warmheartedness Warmth Watchfulness Wealth Willfulness Willingness Winning Wisdom Wittiness Wonder Worthiness Youthfulness Zeal

ABOUT THE AUTHOR

Laurel is a narrative therapist, chronic pain expert and therapeutic innovator who has a private practices in Canada. She started her career in British Columbia working at a drop-in centre with children whose mother's experienced domestic violence. She then became a counsellor at a shelter for women who suffered violence. After that, she worked alongside the Royal Canadian Mounted Police as a victim service advocate, counselling people who lost loved ones to suicide, murder or accidental death. She also works at her community hospital as a Mental Health and Substance Use Counsellor.

Her latest therapeutic innovation titled A Narrative Approach to Dealing with Chronic Pain was recently published in The International Journal of Narrative Therapy and Community Work. She has developed the first narrative therapy chronic pain group in the world and is now sharing this research with therapists in Australia and Singapore.

Laurel holds a Masters degree in Narrative Therapy from the University of Melbourne in Australia and a certificate in Narrative Therapy from the Caspersen Institute through the University of Minnesota. Her bachelor of arts degree is in psychology, and she graduated with honours having received awards in both English and psychology.

Laurel has been working alongside clients experiencing trauma, depression, anxiety, chronic pain, illness, disability,

PTSD and other psychological problems for many years. Her academic studies in psychology and cultural anthropology, together with her personal studies on the work of Joseph Campbell, Michael White, Allan Watts, and of Christianity and Buddhism, have helped shape the approaches she currently uses.

www.ingramcontent.com/pod-product-compliance
Lightning Source LLC
Chambersburg PA
CBHW030733180526
45157CB00008BA/3147